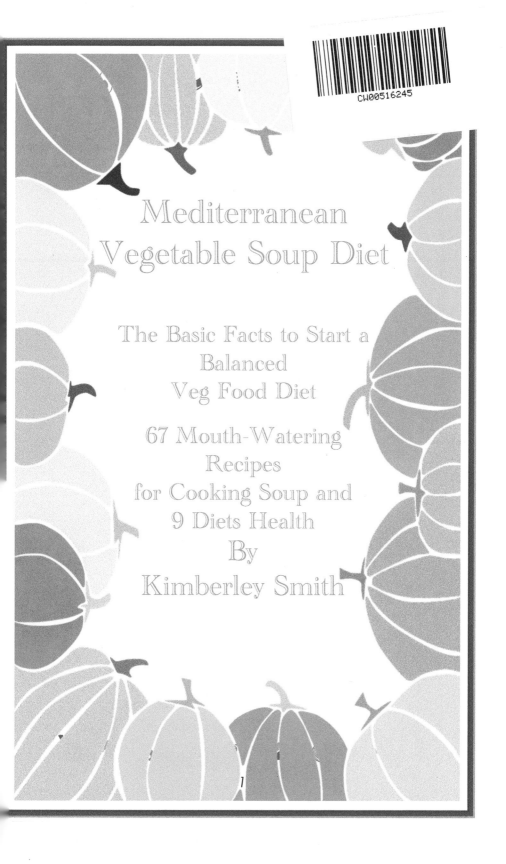

Mediterranean Vegetable Soup Diet

The Basic Facts to Start a Balanced Veg Food Diet

67 Mouth-Watering Recipes for Cooking Soup and 9 Diets Health

By

Kimberley Smith

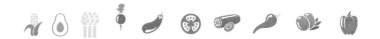

Cover by Bluebird Provisions on Pixabay

Visit the author's page

Write to: kimb.smith.books@gmail.com

OTHER PUBLICATIONS BY KIMBERLEY SMITH:

Raising Chickens For Eggs:

*The Beginner's Guide To Building A Chicken-Coop, To Learn How to Raise A Happy Backyard Flock.
A Homesteading Solution While You Are At Home*

Hydroponic Gardening:

*A Detailed Guide on Hydronics to Learn the Principles Behind Gardening and Build a Wonderful System While at Home.
Techniques for Your Vegetable Cultivations*

Keto Copycat Cookbook Restaurant:

A Keto Diet to Feel Your Best. Easy Recipes for Beginners for All Seasons From Appetizers to Desserts to Reduce Inflammation, Lose Weight, and Heal the Immune System

EASY KETO DESERTS

67 Recipes for Beginners for All Seasons

to Reduce Inflammation, Lose Weight, And Heal the Immune System

A Ketogenic Diet to Feel Your Best

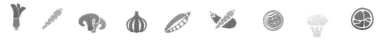

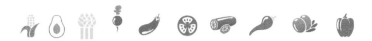

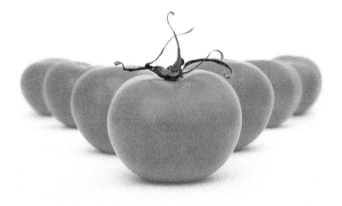

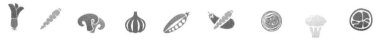

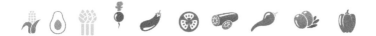

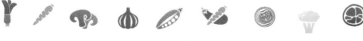

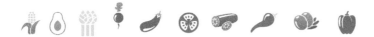

Contents

Vegetarianism and raw food 9

What is raw food? 14

Description and values of vegetarian foods....23

Some diets...45

   Diet for the obese 46

   Diet for the gouty 51

   Diet, for those suffering from eczema 51

   Diabetic diet 52

   Vermifuge diet 52

   Diet for the old men 53

   Diet to gain weight 54

   Diet for constipated 54

   Diet for stomach sufferers 54

Rational way of distributing meals....................56

Cookbook 59

Soups 60

   Neapolitan soup 61

   Portuguese soup 61

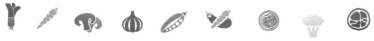

Breadcrumbs Soup   63

Genoese soup   63

Cresa soup 64

Condè Soup   65

Aurora Soup   65

Pseudo-clam soup with marinara   66

Almond soup   67

Pseudo-frog soup 67

Soup of pseudo-clams   68

Celery soup   68

British soap 68

Mountain soup   69

White soup 70

Hard pan soup with tomato   70

Mushroom soup   71

Milk and egg soup   72

Bean soup with celery   72

Italian vegetable soap   72

Pasta with lentils (Soup)   73

Pasta with beans (Soup) 73

Pasta with dried broad beans   74

Pasta with broccoli (Soup)   74

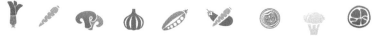

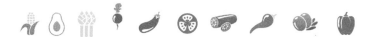

Pasta with green beans   74

Oriental soup   75

Spring soup75

Munich soup   76

Mock-turtle soup   76

Austrian soup   77

Housewife soup   78

Polenta soup with subisso   78

Chilean lentils   79

Maggiolina soup   80

Chilean-style beans   80

Soup house80

Breaded soup   81

Sour Potato Soup   82

Passatelle in Italian-style soup   82

Duxellese soup   83

Green soup   84

Varied green soup   84

London soup   85

Julian soup 85

English macaroni soup   86

Leek soup   86

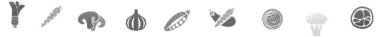

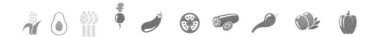

Egyptian lens soup   87

Soup of lentils and rice   87

English milk soup   87

Mushroom soup   88

Ricotta soup   89

Winter Soup   89

Chilean Puchero   90

Rumford Soup   91

White beans soup 91

Green soup   91

Raw soups 93

Soup with Corn   94

Raw spring soup   94

Winter soup95

Cantaloupe soup   95

Beetroot soup   96

Semolina soup   96

Spicy soup for stomach dullers   96

Soup with corn   97

Fresh tomato soup97

Soup of cereals and dried legumes   98

Complete tomato soap   99

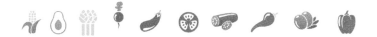

Vegetarianism and raw food

Let us first examine the proper and etymological meaning of the word vegetarianism.

Derived from the verb vegetate, it serves to define that lifestyle considered to be the most rational for making the human body vegetarian.

Therefore, it is not limited only to the nourishment of the latter, but to everything that contributes to the perfect success of its vegetative process.

To a regime of life of an ethical and prophylactic nature equally pure and in harmony with the laws of Nature.

Man, through centuries of prejudice and abuse, has transpired the true origin of him who is eminently fugacious as his teeth also testify.

The slow atavistic degeneration that has ensued has meant that his maximum life span, which (as recognized by science) should reach 130 years, reaches just half an average.

It is a mistake to believe that he can no longer go back and restore his original regime without suffering at least momentary disturbances.

Maybe the transition from a carnivorous regime to a strictly vegetarian one, with only cooked vegetables, can cause transient and never serious disturbances, but the transition to a naturalistic, or

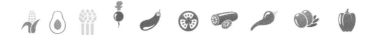

even better raw, regime is a true liberation and an absolute regenerating purification.

Moreover, due to excessive prudence, it can also be done gradually and progressively.

For man's nourishment, the following basic elements are necessary: proteins, carbohydrates, mineral salts, fats, cellulose, vitamins, etc.

Now Nature lavishes us all this spontaneously and directly from wheat fields to colorful orchards, from verdant vegetable gardens to flowery prairies where the cow and the hen joyfully draw the elements to give us the milk that is surplus to one from the nutrition of its young and the eggs that overabound the other in proportion to its possibilities of brooding.

Man, with the abuse of his freedom of action on animals, has dissociated this power of will from his responsibility of conscience on which he depends.

The best way to live in harmony is, reclaiming the earth by cultivating it and working it constantly and by presiding over it; the beasts, reptiles, and all animals, plants, and herbs of lower evolutionary cycles will not be able to live there, while life will thus be forced to flow in forms of higher evolution; rationally build your homes, take care of the hygiene of your body with maximum cleanliness, laborious life, purely natural food, upright and sober mental conduct, and life through the lower forms of insects, parasites, microbes, etc., will not be able to develop around you.

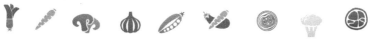

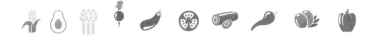

By transgressing all these precise and unchanging, and therefore inexorable laws, man has reduced the period of his natural existence and has made each of his bodily life a real burden of ailments.

He has hindered the great plan of evolution, sacrifying the young sensitive lives of the animals, which he must instead perfect and advance.

Medical science, is forced to limit its work to the sole treatment of the ailments already done and we see climatic stations, health resorts, dietary establishments, etc., spring up every moment; all with more or less vegetarian treatments depending on the possibility of readiness to adapt.

However, late repairs can only stop the continuation of the destructive work, and what has been destroyed can no longer be rebuilt.

Therefore, all that remains is to cry the alarm so that we can retrace our steps to regain that long and healthy life, the bearer of happiness, which is the heritage of man.

In the vegetarian, naturist regime, in addition to having healthy and pure food, we find everything that can satisfy the most refined tastes.

A plate of pasta topped with cheese and butter, and some fruit, alone would represent all the nutrition that man needs; therefore, one should not renounce to pleasure of the table.

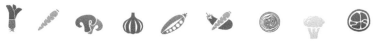

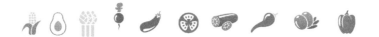

The incentive to restore the body, with a sober meal, must coincide with the restoration of the mind.

Thus, the physiological restorative action of the body is not completed, it must not be an end in itself, that is, a gross material enjoyment, but it must be a means to return small new energies to the heart so that the spirit can, through this instrument put in order, make them all flow.

Active vegetative life and thinking spiritual life are the two inseparable expressions of the Spirit who realizes his being in this synthesis.

Although man may fell full, even with a handful of seeds and fruit, he must not give up, when he can, at lunchtime which, even if modest, represents in our life a moment of upright and healthy joy; in which the entire harmony of forces and feelings is restored and exalted.

You cannot eat and assimilate food well if you do not enjoy peace and joy and you cannot be happy if you do not nourish yourself healthily, measuredly with pure foods.

"Mens sana in corpore sano"

The theory of the old biological school advocates that from meat we can draw certain amino acids, while we cannot find them directly in the vegetable kingdom. This is refuted by the facts that have always practically proved how man not only could live but lives better only with the products of the earth.

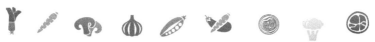

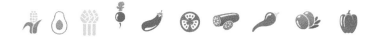

On the other hand, it is enough to empirically observe that the animals, whose meat has been studied and in whose meat amino acids have been found, are exclusively herbivores.

Now if they can carry out this elaborative process through the food of herbs only, in a better way it will be able to disengage a higher-order organism through a complete naturist diet.

Therefore, the alleged usefulness and even less the alleged need to resort to lazy and degrading parasitism not worthy of the nobility of the human being, both as an ethical individuality and as a biological entity, does not hold up.

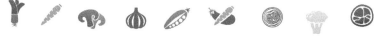

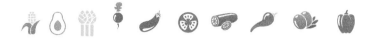

What is raw food?

We have entertained ourselves and have provided abundant formulas for all those who, while wanting to make a very useful effort with eliminating necrophagy, still hold and are still attached to all the scaffolding and artificial gear of kitchen, cooks, dishwashers, pots, dishes, banquets, and all that is used for nothing other than to waste money and human activities, which could much more profitably be employed in works useful for the evolutionary ascension of humanity.

But there is an even better way to free yourself not only from the burden of cooking, cooked and feasted but from the efforts to which our organism undergoes to transform and assimilate cooked foods and animal products, even if they are not meat products. It is the regime based on everything that nature offers us, not altered by cooking.

Although many chemical combinations that occur during cooking have not yet been specified, it is certain, however, that in addition to killing some vitamins and diastases, acids, salts, etc. are severely altered and all the vital efficiencies that have now been recognized by science are not only useful but necessary for the regular functioning and immunization of our organism.

Sugar, for example, which in its natural state can be found in fruit, milk, and some roots, combined with acids and salts, is of great nutritional and energetic

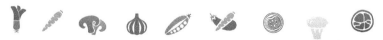

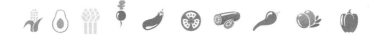

value, very easy to be burnt by our body; while after being cooked and neutralized by industry, it becomes so inert that it cannot even be transformed by saccharomyces.

Our organism struggles enormously to reverse it and burn it because it must first reoxidize it with gastric acids to return it in part to the state as it is found in nature.

Often and in the long run, our organism does not have the resources and the strength to carry out this tiring recovery and the neutral sugar passes unnoticed into the blood causing diabetes and other serious imbalances and pathological changes.

Let's see how the tomato, which in its raw state is a dissolver, diuretic, vitalizing, digestive and refreshing; after cooked, on the other hand, it becomes perfectly the opposite, determining uric acids, liver stones, warming form of the viscera and urinary tract, indigestible, and loses all vitalizing power.

These still mysterious powers, of which science has recently come to discover some, are not limited only to these, and we can have proof of them through personal observation.

Let's see for example fish in an aquarium that lives perfectly if the water is constantly renewed with other water drawn from the sea or from a source of the earth, but if you stop this exchange, after 24 hours they begin to deteriorate and then die, even if

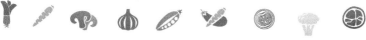

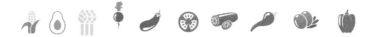

you give them some food that can make up for those substances contained in running water.

There is therefore a vitalizing factor in the products of the earth in the living state which is neither substance nor vitamin, nor diastasis, but of equal maximum importance whose nature we do not yet know.

But for now, it is enough for us to know only the effects to be able to regulate our eating behavior and we will call this factor: Biogenin x.

Many illustrious scientists such as the Lehmann's, Cristen, Carton, Bircher, Benner, Bachman, Drews, Haig, Bienstock, Tomson, Gerson, Muësle, and many others, have obtained remarkable results both in terms of therapy and prophylactic prevention against ailments, and in fact, while the healings are innumerable, the resistance as prevention to all diseases (not due to ethical errors) can be said to be absolute.

In this regard, it is good to clarify this distinction.

All the diseases that afflict humanity (which should leave the body only for the serene extinction of old age) come from two great causes: ethical error and dietary error.

They determine the pathological effect both in the person who makes the mistake and in his descendants. The best way to cope with it is the development of individual understanding.

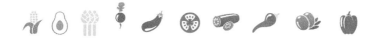

Therefore, it is enough for us to deal with the dietary error, while for the other each one will provide for himself through his own experiences and knowledge.

Our being in harmony with ethical laws and not disturbed by irrational nutrition is perfectly resistant to any external attack.

Distracting his resistances by forcing him to laborious digestions and continued detoxification puts him in conditions of leaving place to the attacks of inferior organic lives, which only in this way can take over and undermine their regular functioning of our organism.

In addition to this, the impossibility of completely freeing oneself from all the toxic substances ingested causes a slow and progressive accumulation of poisons that increases over and over, with the decreasing of the elimination powers as time goes by.

If some consequences of a mis correct diet can therefore be solved when in younger age, it is fatal it is fatal for the elderly.

With the raw naturist regime in harmony with the so-called ethics, true liberation from all evils is obtained.

We know that the elements necessary for our nutrition are: proteins, hydrocarbons, mineral salts, fats, cellulose, and vital efficiencies (those known under the name of vitamins and diastase) and those

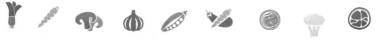

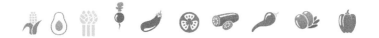

known under the name of biogenous what nature lavishes on us in vegetables, fruit, seeds, milk, and eggs, and hands them to us so skillfully combined, that any modification that man wants to make on them can only damage them.

Therefore, having left the task of elaborating them to nature, all that remains for man is to know how to use them, and even in this, the wise nature gives us the means with the alternatives of the seasons. In any case, we give a schematic picture of the powers of vegetable foods that can be eaten raw, so that the reader can make his own food behavior.

It is good to remind that protein or albumin is commonly called no more than a 1 oz. to 50 per day, what is found in 3,5 oz. in oil seeds or in in a cup of milk or an egg.

Then come the hydrocarbons and fats.

The latter can be increased especially in winter to give more calories, with olive oil and butter.

All the rest, mineral salts, cellulose, and vital efficiencies of all kinds can be found both in seeds and in raw vegetables and fruit.

In my opinion, the very shredding and handling of such things should be avoided.

You see the goat, the rabbit, the gazelle, which refuse even the most tender buds simply because they have been touched by man.

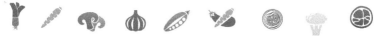

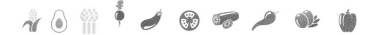

Vegetables bought at the market should be revived in running water, fruit equally, oilseeds, peel them off when eating them, and having good teeth avoid mechanical grinding.

However, for those who still care about going to the table, the portions and the aesthetics of the same, as for those whose dentition no longer helps them to chew the seeds, we suggest some formulas based on which they can make an infinity of them.

The interesting and essential thing is to know that a handful of oilseeds, a handful of cereals or legumes macerated in water and a couple of pounds of assorted vegetables and fruit is all that is not only enough for us to nourish ourselves well, but it feeds us most appropriately. rational, hygienic, and prophylactic.

To make raw food combinations, it is first of all necessary to thoroughly clean both the tools and the vegetables and herbs themselves, which must always be washed with running water.

It is also necessary to have a lemon squeezer, a rasping machine, a grater for oilseeds, a squeezer and grinder, and a mortar, possibly in porcelain.

Specific properties of some vegetables

Sweet almonds, in addition to being a complete food because they contain carbohydrates, proteins, fats, mineral salts, cellulose, and a large number of vital efficiencies, if well peeled by keeping them in

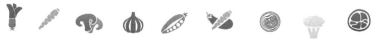

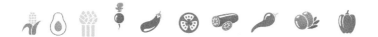

fresh water (never hot because it destroys a large part of vital efficiencies) and well minced, are of a great balsamic and refreshing action for stomach patients (you must avoid bitter ones, which instead are harmful for your health, so you have to taste them one by one).

Plums, even dried ones, macerated in freshwater, are laxative and therefore very suitable for constipation by adjusting the daily quantity according to your body.

Since their action is also refreshing, they can be taken in very large quantities in order to obtain the desired effect without any harmful consequences, as it happens with drugs.

Garlic, in addition to being full of vital efficiencies, while raw is a powerful disinfectant of the gastric passages.

The radishes are excellent dissolvers of stones and urates.

Carrots, like onions, are mineralizing and vitalizing elements per excellence. Parsley has a powerful regulating action on the circulation and replacement of the blood.

Sugary fruits are energetic and refreshing, so when you are very tired it is very suitable to take dates, raisins, bananas, figs, etc., drinking a good almond juice or coconut juice over them.

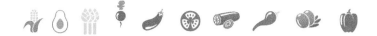

All the organic acids of fruit are extremely precious as diuretic dissolvents, stimulants, and compensators: the malic acid of the apple, the tartaric acid of the grapes, the citric acid of the citrus fruits, the quinic of the cherries and sour cherries, etc.

They also contain pectin, which transforms the organic juices of the fruits into jelly.

All vegetables, such as spinach, lettuce, etc., and also the roots, in addition to the other mineral salts, also contain sodium chloride (cooking salt) in a proportion sufficient to supply the small losses we have; for which it is necessary to make use of very small doses of cooking salt, even being able to do without it, having proved that salt beyond this small requirement is harmful.

If you eat oil seeds youdo not need cereals, but if you want to add them to meals, you can use them by soaking them in water until they become soft up to the center; then they are rinsed in fresh water, ground in the grinder, and seasoned with shaved roots, chopped vegetables, garlic, onion, oil, and lemon, thus obtaining dishes rich in energy and support for the hardest physical efforts. For mental fatigue, a few raw oilseeds are enough to repair the phosphorus loss.

It is a great mistake to worry about typhus bacilli, meba, or others that can be found in raw vegetables, because the bacilli cannot penetrate

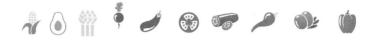

the living tissues of the plants, but only remain outside and therefore are easily eliminated with a good washing.

If you want to do naturism for therapeutic purposes, it is good to completely omit common salt (sodium chloride) and replace it with celery salt.

All raw cucurbits well-chewed or chopped have a special cleansing and refreshing action on the intestinal mucous membranes as well as forming an excellent push move for the expulsion of feces

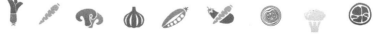

Description and values of vegetarian foods

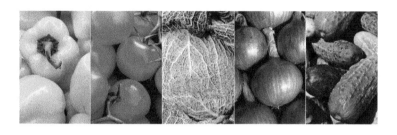

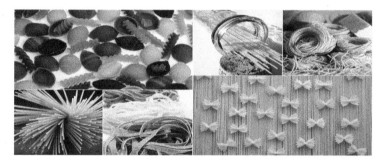

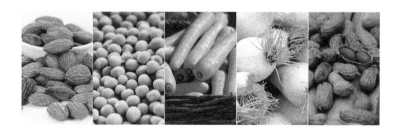

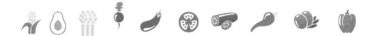

Cereals. *This family is made up of six grains: wheat, rye, oats, barley, rice, and corn, represents the most important part of human food.*

Wheat. *It stands at the head of others for its content in gluten, vitamins, nitrogenous substances; carbohydrates and mineral salts. It is actually nourishment of primary importance also for its cheapness.*

Bread, which is the best handling of wheat, has been the subject of endless discussions for choosing the best way to work it.

We do not dwell on mentioning the many opinions, almost all of which are extremist, but we only say our opinion on the subject, which lies in a middle way.

Since gluten and vitamins are adherents to the woody integument that covers the grain of wheat, it is recommended to make whole bread (with all the bran) to have all the gluten and all the vitamins.

Now as a little inert mass is useful for the catabolism process and a little less gluten and vitamins do not greatly diminish the nutritional values, we believe that the most convenient is a bread that is not completely made by whole meal, a brown bread, that is, reduced to 82%, exactly what our farmers do, whose centuries-old experience and taste, specialized for the most part on this food, have led them to this proportion.

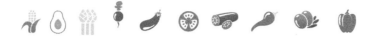

Pasta. *(another derivative of wheat). With this name, we mean all types of macaroni, spaghetti, lasagna, etc., etc. seasoned in various ways as it is practiced in all countries of the world.*

This excellent and popular food occupies a place of primary importance in vegetarian cuisine, both for its mild cost, suitable for all bags, and its great nutritional value.

Given the infinite variety of flavors to which it can be brought, you can eat it all the days of the year and all the years of life, without ever getting tired.

It is very easy to prepare there is no woman at home who in half an hour does not know how to prepare an excellent dish of dry pasta or soup.

A plate of pasta, topped with cheese and butter or with any sauce, is the complete food par excellence, and cheaper than any other.

Wheat provides it with carbohydrates, gluten, protein, and cellulose, while butter gives it fat and aroma, and cheese another protein which, combined with that of wheat, completes it by the difference of specific characters, also giving it another kind of vivifying and energetic elements and completing its flavor.

The variation of sauces and condiments alternates the differences of the aforesaid elements thus facilitating their daily digestion.

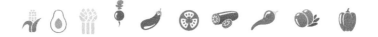

Its way of cooking it (especially in southern Italy), that is, in a lot water, then separating it from the latter, makes it much lighter, melted, and therefore more digestible; because some salts difficult to be affected by gastric juices are diluted in the water in which it boils, and a certain amount of starchy substances is also released, thus reducing its composition to a more balanced and more assimilable complex.

Pasta is unjustly infamous as a fattening agent, while this power takes it only from the toxic substances of meat and animal fats with which it is seasoned or combined during the meal and of which it is only a vehicle.

You see, for example, all the peasants of Sicily who daily eat pasta seasoned only with olive oil, or cheese, or tomato, without adding or combining it with meat or animal fats; they are all dry temperatures of very strong fiber resistant to the heaviest work under the lash of the sun or the harsh winter.

They do not know what they are: obesity, fatness, while as soon as we go up to the more comfortable classes, where the first luxury you have is to eat a second dish of meat or season the pasta with sausage, minced meat, clams, and animal fats, we immediately see the fatness, obesity and all their serious consequences, settling in those organisms.

Pasta, eaten in the right quantity alone or accompanied by strictly vegetable and raw second courses, is not fattening at all, being assimilated and ready to be replaced due to the ease of digestion; in the same way as pure water cannot be fatty when taken alone on an empty stomach, and which instead becomes fatty if ingested during meals based on meat and animal fats.

By the same fact it becomes its vehicle, increasing the action of fats on the proliferation of fat cells which are always growing, especially with advancing age; in which the necessarily more sedentary life and the natural slowing down of the replacement powers favor these accumulations of fat.

Rye. It comes immediately after wheat due to the nutritional value of its substance and is, however, less rich in starchy matter and with a particularly pleasant taste, it is used to mix with wheat to obtain a lighter, tastier, and more durable bread.

By itself, for the same reasons, it is food for diabetics and sick people, lighter than wheat.

Barley. This cereal, very rich in mucilaginous materials, is excellent for nutritional decoctions, for the convalescents and children.

Because of these qualities, it was always used in family therapy, even as an emollient and laxative, since the time of Hippocrates who prescribed it, especially in his care.

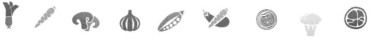

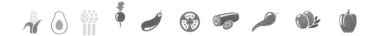

Oat. Both in the form of flour and displacement, as they are widely used in England (Quaker-Oats), it constitutes a food very rich in salts and phosphorus and very easy to digest, so it is indicated for food for children, old people, and of those who work a lot mentally.

It is prepared in puree, in decoction, or soup with milk. Quaker-Oats is now also prepared in Italy in boxes with instructions for use.

Used raw and marinated in water for 12 hours is even better.

Rice. It is the poorest of cereals in nitrogenous substances and the richest in carbohydrates.

It would be a food of great value, but the industrialization of it, to make it white and shiny by decorticating and bleaching, takes away the most important elements: the mineral, diastatic, nitrogenous principles and vitamins, reducing it to a simple dead starch.

Brown rice is now on the market and its use is highly recommended almost like that of wheat.

Corn. It is also an excellent nutrient.

There are regions where the peasants can be said to live on corn only in the form of poultry; in South America, it is used in the form of cornstarch, that is, first roasted and then milled in impalpable flour.

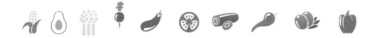

This is the best way to use it because it is dextrinized so it is easier to digest and has a delicious taste, especially in the manufacture of biscotti and sweets.

Spoiled corn causes pellagra.

The eggs. This product that nature lavishes on us with superabundance, since, especially the hen, produces it far beyond its possibilities of reproduction, is evidently destined for human nutrition.

Prepared for the construction of a complete animal organism, it contains all the basic elements for the life of the future organism, so we draw from it in a very small volume, a perfect complex of nutritional, energetic, and vitalizing substances.

Its weight is on average 2 oz. of which, removed the shell, 1,2 oz consist of white and 6 oz. from the yolk.

The egg white contains for the most part proteins, iron, and silica; the red part, instead, is richer in nitrogen materials, phosphorus, lecithin, fats, energy materials, and vitamins. A food of this value must be the restorative basis of convalescents and growing children.

From one to three egg yolks a day constitute a regenerating nourishment par excellence and this maximum number must not be exceeded, which however must always be combined with fruit, vegetables, and seeds.

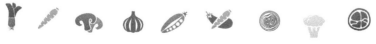

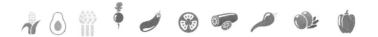

Legumes. In them, we also find all the constituents of meat with the addition of carbohydrates, mineral salts, vitamins, and other positive substances, while they are free of all the toxic substances that are additionally found in meat.

At the forefront are lentils with 26% albumin and 59% carbohydrates; then the peas with 24% and 62% respectively, then the beans, chickpeas, broad beans, etc.

However, dried legumes, unlike cereals, contain mineral salts, especially in the woody casing, which, due to their being of little soluble nature, can therefore be difficult to digest, causing special flatulence if taken in large quantities and with all the skins.

This does not happen, however, when they are still green, especially peas, which in this state are highly digestible by the most sickly stomachs, as well as being of exquisite flavor.

To help dissolve the insoluble salts of dried legumes, bicarbonate of soda is excellent, putting a pinch of it during cooking, as well as passing them through a sieve, to separate them from the woody integument.

Mushrooms and truffles. It is worth talking about it in isolation because this family of vegetables, so distinctly original in all its characteristics, is also endowed with very marked nutritional values.

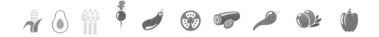

They contain from 20 to 25% albumin mixed with abundant mineral salts and cellulose. In a limited volume, they are therefore very useful and deliciously flavored food.

The truffle, however, being very concentrated and expensive, must be used in moderation and only as a condiment.

Regarding mushrooms, there are many poisonous varieties, but the naturalist Nessler states that, since mushroom poison is a soluble narcotic in sodium chloride (kitchen salt) and acetic acid, immersing them for a few hours in a saltwater solution with wine vinegar, the poisonous substances dissolve remaining in the solution. By repeatedly rinsing the mushrooms in freshwater, they would remain perfectly harmless.

He says that he and his family ate the most poisonous qualities treated in this way for an entire month.

In any case, just eat those well-known local qualities or those produced by artificial crops, which are now found everywhere and which are very safe.

All those alleged tests of the little women: that of the coin, the silver fork, etc., are all to be banned because traces of hydrogen sulfide are enough to make the silver blacken, without the mushrooms being poisonous at all, or vice versa, there may be poisonous mushrooms which do not blacken the silver because not containing the aforesaid acid.

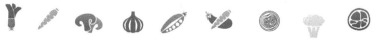

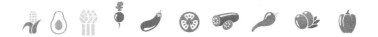

The milk. This food, also supplied to us by nature with superabundance, since, especially the cow, produces much more of it than the needs of its calves, it is also of precious importance.

It contains proteins, a sugar called lactose, mineral salts, and vital efficiencies. All in a stable emulsion and therefore very easy to assimilate.

Very rich in calcium, it is a precious food for children by helping bone formation.

For the milk to be in its full nutritional and vitalizing completeness, it must be taken as soon as it is fed, while all its dynamogenic properties and biogenesis are in full efficiency. It must be ensured that the animal is not sick and its udders must be thoroughly cleaned before being milked and so must the milker's hands.

Milk should also be avoided when it contains colostrum, that is in the first days after childbirth, which is easy to recognize by the yellow color it presents.

Boiled milk loses all its vital powers and diastasis, so it remains a stunted food, limited only to casein and butter; it is, therefore, useful, only for cooking, completing it with other ingredients, or for making cheese, or for a partially nutritious drink to be completed with other things in vital efficiency (fruit, vegetables, etc.).

Butter.

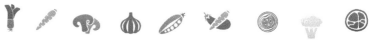

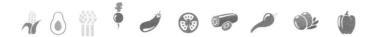

Produced from pure cream, or cream, or mozzarella if you prefer, in the raw state it is a very light and digestible fat, because it derives from a stable emulsion, such as milk, and therefore it's very easy to be re emulsified by biliary secretion and then digested immediately.

Without being cooked, it contains large quantities of diastase and vitamins, so it is advisable to use it at the table by putting it in dishes at the time of eating or, better still, eating it on bread as an appetizer or intermediary.

To take advantage of its vitalizing powers and its aromatic qualities, in addition to the raw state, it must be fresh and pure cream.

The cheese.

It is derived from curdled milk from which the watery part can thus be removed while maintaining, in a compacted mass, all the nitrogenous material emulsified with the butter.

Thus it is also a food very rich in proteins, fat, calcium salts, and abundant diastases.

Creamy or double cream cheeses are excellent and very nutritious because cream removed from other milk was added to the milk before curdling it; then come the whole cheeses, that is, to which no cream has been removed or added, then low-fat cheeses

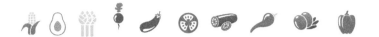

that are those whose milk has been removed from the cream to make butter.

It goes without saying that the former have a nutritious superiority, that the latter is excellent, and that the thirds can be used for condiments. In all cases, the so-called strong fermented cheeses due to their strong spicy taste are to be outlawed.

The fermentation microbes transform albumin into leucine, tyrosine, ammonium carbonate, fats into fatty acids and develop toxic-aromatic substances which, due to their stimulating power, appeal to degenerate tastes; in the same way as you can enjoy the salivating stimulus of the nicotine of tobacco.

All the products of the fermentation of cheese and which are the beginning of real putrefaction, are harmful and poisonous. It is easy to recognize unfermented cheeses first by their good smell, then by their light color, by the compact mass without veins or greenish grinds where real molds are collected with species of granules that are nothing more than worm eggs to be found in a second period of corruption.

Ricotta.

This other derivative of milk is also an extremely important food; it must be fresh, one or two days at the most and it is easy to recognize it because as soon as it is altered it immediately takes on an acrid odor and acid taste.

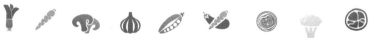

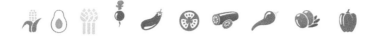

It contains all the substances of cheese, but with a much lower proportion of casein and therefore it is much easier to digest.

With it, infinite qualities of dishes and desserts are prepared, all very nutritious, light, and exquisite.

The oils and fats.

First of all, there is the pure olive oil of the highest quality, that is the one extracted from the mature olive harvested from the tree and which must therefore not exceed 2% acidity.

The olive oil that has fallen and dried on the ground, like that of the stone, must be discarded.

The first is a fat of the highest order due to its lightness and finesse given to it by the vegetable processing.

Besides having a very delicate fruit taste, it is very easy to be emulsified by the biliary juice and therefore easy to digest and completely assimilate; contains glycerin which makes it an excellent lubricant for the digestive tract.

Peanut, sesame, cotton, and other seed oils, when well refined, are also excellent fats for cooking, but it is advisable to combine them with olive oil or butter because, being neutral in taste, they need the sapidity that can be given to them by the latter.

Coconut fat is also excellent for cooking alone.

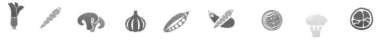

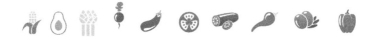

It is also edible raw mixed with the butter from which it takes the aroma.

All animal fats, due to their weight greater than that of vegetable fats and butter and the difficulty of being emulsified by bile, are difficult to digest, in addition to their more or less nauseating taste.

They contain some of the toxins of meat and are easy, due to the difficult digestive processing, to act directly on the proliferation of fat cells, thus promoting obesity.

Salads and vegetables.

Especially those that can be ingested raw are of great importance in the economy of our organism; in the raw state, they are very rich in vitamins and salts and are a vitalizing element par excellence and dissolving acids and toxins.

Cellulose, which is the main part of their construction, is necessary to constitute the mechanical mass that exerts pressure against the walls of the intestine, causing its peristaltic activity.

Thus the process of catabolism and the expulsion of digestive waste are favored, avoiding stagnation and the consequent absorption of toxins.

The danger of infectious diseases is a prejudice since when our organism is in conditions of attack, it will always and everywhere find enemies ready to attack it, whether it eats raw vegetables or not.

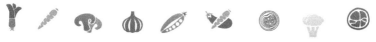

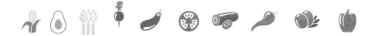

With the vegetable regime and healthy life, physically and ethically, the bacilli, which can be found both in raw vegetables and on any other food, on the edge of a glass where a fly has simply placed bread touched by infected fingers, will be attacked and destroyed by our natural defenses, which have not been exhausted and weakened by the laborious digestion of meat foods, which constitute a true environment of bacterial culture.

The salt

(chemically sodium chloride) is contained in our organism and it was therefore considered useful to supply it again in those small doses with which it is lost.

Exaggerating its use, it becomes irritating to the kidneys and mucous membranes of the intestine.

Celery salt is much more hygienic.

Aromas and spices.

In small and non-continuous doses, they are useful elements not only for the good taste of dishes but for the stimulation of gastric secretions and peristaltic movements.

By exaggerating their use, they are irritating, inflammatory and can produce serious disorders of the urinary and gastric tract.

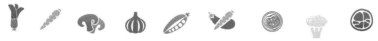

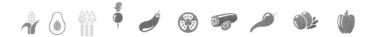

Most harmful of all is black or white pepper, while cayenne and mustard are stronger but far less irritating. However, it is better to make as little use as possible.

The sugar.

This energetic element par excellence, concentrated in a very small volume, gives the greatest number of calories, absorbing itself very quickly without leaving any waste residue.

A small quantity of it ingested after a great effort is enough to immediately restore energy.

However, there is a big difference, to be taken into account, between inactive, neutralized sugar, in short, rendered inert by commercial manufacture and sugar supplied to us directly by nature through fruit, roots, milk, honey, etc.; this, inactive combination with mineral salts and diastases loaded with vitamins, is much more energetic, vitalizing and easier to be burned.

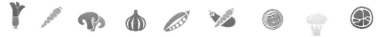

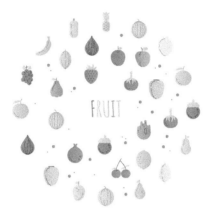

Fresh fruit and oily fruit.

Fresh fruit, and oily fruit (walnuts, almonds, hazelnuts, peanuts, pistachios, pine nuts, etc.), as we have already said, are in their entirety the complete and most rational food for man.

All nutritional elements are contained in their totality: proteins, carbon hydrates, fats, mineral salts, cellulose, vitamins, and biogenies.

Fresh fruits, with soft pulp, well ripe, are an ace, a true detoxifying and vitalizing food.

They are very suitable for feverish patients.

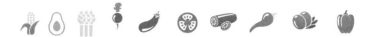

It is advisable to eat fruit with the peel when this is very thin and you are sure you can macerate it well with careful chewing.

Fruits are also very useful as repairers of the brain due to the considerable quantities of nitrogen and phosphoric acid they contain and are also precious for the dissolution of uric acids, due to the abundant potassium salts and organic acids they contain.

The vitamins.

This active principle, of supreme and necessary importance in the economy of our organism, was known by ancient Eastern wisdom under the Sanskrit generic term of Prana and experimental science, in its tireless investigative work to discern the truth from the imposture, into which ancient occult knowledge fell in the Middle Ages, has been able today experimentally ascertain the existence of this active principle in food and its indispensability in nutrition, because it is life.

Up to now, 5 classes of vitamins have been established, specifying them with the alphabetic letters A, B, C, D, E.

This denomination was given for the first time by Funk, in 1911 and the classifications by letters were given according to where they were extracted from and their specific characteristics.

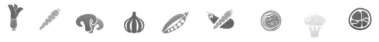

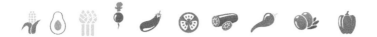

Thus the vitamins isolated in the green part of vegetables, in milk, butter, and egg yolk were classified with the letter A.

They resist cooking and their lack of food causes developmental disorders, cachexia, rachitis.

Those with the letter B are found in the woody integument of cereals, in fresh and dried vegetables, also in milk, yeast, and bread; they resist the long boiling and their absence causes slimming, the beriberi of the Chinese (peeled rice eaters), and other serious disorders of the nervous system.

Those classified with the letter C are found in fresh vegetables, in fruit, also in milk, in whole eggs, and especially in citrus fruit juice.

They are sterilized by cooking.

Their absence generates scurvy, Barlow's disease, and other unspecified ailments.

While their absence causes such serious consequences, their presence stimulates nitrogen exchange and generates vital energies.

Vitamins D, are essential to avoid demineralization and therefore premonitory tuberculosis, chronic rheumatism, descaling menopause, etc.

Vitamins E, in abundance in wheat, lettuce, cabbage, etc., are very useful for growth and reproduction.

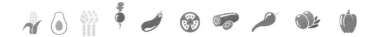

All other vital efficiencies not yet identified we will call them biogenic x.

Herbal teas.

They are divided into two categories: Infusions and decoctions.

For the former, lemon, tea, coffee, lime, chamomile, orange blossom, cedar, mandarin, lime, bitter orange, etc. are used.

They are prepared by pouring boiling water over the product from which the active yield is to be obtained.

Decoctions are formed with roots, vegetables, cocoa, lichens, quinine, pigeon, laurel, thyme, mallow, weed, wormwood, dried fruit, etc., whose values we will talk about later.

Raw infusions are also made in order not to kill the biogenic x

The drinks.

Excluding all those with alcoholic compounds, we can make them in large quantities with the sauce of all fruits starting with lemon, oranges, and other citrus fruits, which are all of a great value, and ending with the nutritious, milky ones extracted from sweet almonds, coconut, from barley, etc.

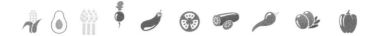

They are all useful both as dissolvents, in a healthy state of health, and as repairers in case of illness, when one cannot or must not eat.

Wine (it is the derivative of one of the best and most useful products of the vegetable kingdom which is grapes).

One of its components, sugar, is transformed into alcohol (due to the work of the bacteria called saccharomyces).

Our palate suggests and searches for a fine and very aged wine, which can be recognized by the delicious natural scent it emanates.

This comes from the fact that the alcohol in contact with the wine acids slowly transforms itself into ethers.

It is known how medicine uses commercial ethers (which is much less than the natural ethers of wine) to lift the organism and make it overcome the moment of crisis.

A few sips of excellent old wine, therefore, helps digestion and is an element of savings.

Vinegar.

Alcohol from wine to another bacteria, mycoderma-vinegar, is transformed into acetic acid.

It is deleterious and poisonous in our organism and its use must be forbidden except in cooking because, being the acetic acid volatilizable to boiling, put in

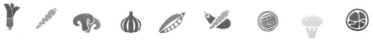

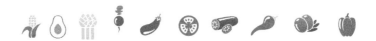

a small quantity in cooked dishes, it preserves only the aromatic part, which is not harmful.

In salads, it is, therefore, preferable to use lemon, which instead gives them the freshness of taste and vitalizing energies.

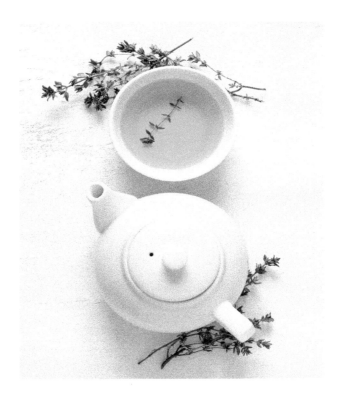

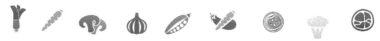

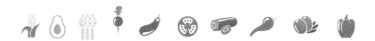

Some diets

These diets are recommendations, so you should consult your doctor before starting the diet

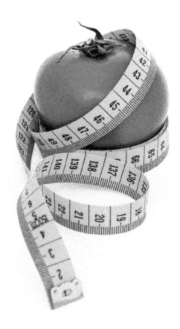

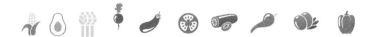

Diet for the obese

Obesity is an imbalance of exchange due in large part to proper or atavic dietary errors for which it is by modifying the causes that the best results are obtained.

The obese must certainly resort to the following raw naturism:

The organism rationally and without problems

The patient must strictly adhere to the following treatment if he really wants to put his organism ruined by obesity in order.

With this diet, which is the synthesis of years of study, he will have surprising results and without any suffering, he will decrease in 18 days of treatment, from 11 to 33 lb.

The sense of well-being, lightness, agility, and good humor immediately comes from it.

Leading precisely to a true renewal and rejuvenation of the whole being.

First day

Morning: 1/2 grapefruit or an orange or 1 lemon sliced with honey, an egg (Possibly raw with lemon juice, salt, and mustard if you like, or boiled to the point you want), a slice of toast, ½ lettuce, tea, coffee without sugar or milk.

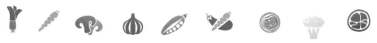

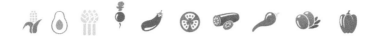

Evening: Unfermented cheese 2,5 oz., 6 slices watermelon, ½ grapefruit, or orange or 1 lemon sliced with honey, tea, or coffee.

Second day

Morning: Two oranges or 2,20 lb. of watermelon, 1 egg, a slice of toast, 2 lettuce, tea, or coffee.

Evening: 2 eggs, a lettuce heart or 4 roots, a tomato or an apple, an orange or ½ grapefruit, tea or coffee without sugar or milk.

Third day

Morning: 2 grapefruit or an orange or 2,20 lb. of watermelon, one egg, 4 raw artichoke hearts, or 8 slices of watermelon, tea, or coffee.

Evening: Fresh cheese 2,5 oz., an egg, 3 radishes, or a cabbage 4 olives, tea, or coffee without sugar or milk.

Fourth day

Morning: 2 eggs, a slice of toast, a tomato or an apple, or 2 raw artichokes, ½ grapefruit or an orange, tea or coffee.

Evening: 8.50 fl. oz. (US) of whole milk, 4 sugar-free biscuits, an orange or 2 grapefruit, tea or coffee without sugar or milk.

Fifth day

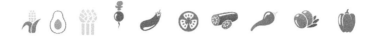

Morning: An orange or 2,20 lb. of watermelon, one egg, 4 olives, tea or coffee.

Evening: Fresh cheese, a slice of toast, 8 slices of cocoa or 2 apples, an orange, tea or coffee without sugar or milk.

Sixth day

Morning: Fresh cheese, 2 tomatoes or 2 artichokes or 4 raw roots, 2 melons or watermelon or 2 oranges, tea or coffee.

Evening: one egg, 3 radishes, 2 tomatoes or 2 sour apples, 6 slices of watermelon or 2 hearts of lettuce, tea or coffee without sugar or milk.

Seventh day

Morning: 2 eggs, a tomato or a sour apple, a slice of toast, ½ melon or 2 pears, tea or coffee.

Evening: An orange, fresh cheese, honey with 2 biscuits, a raw pepper or 2 raw artichokes or 2 lettuce hearts, tea or coffee without sugar or milk.

Eighth day

Morning: An egg, 4 olives, 10 slices of watermelon or 2 sour apples, 2 grapefruit or an orange, tea or coffee without sugar or milk.

Evening: Fresh cheese, a slice of toast, a tomato or an apple, 2 oranges, tea, or coffee without sugar or milk.

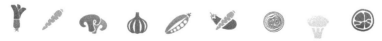

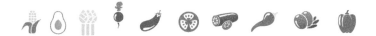

Ninth day

Morning: 12 well-chewed raw almonds or hazelnuts, a pepper or 3 raw artichokes or two cabbage, 6 slices of watermelon or 2 sour apples, an orange or ½ grapefruit, tea or coffee without sugar or milk.

Evening: An egg, tomato, or an apple, 3 roots, lemon with honey, ½ melon or watermelon or two oranges, tea or coffee without sugar or milk.

Day 10

Morning: 2 eggs, a slice of toast, 6 olives, an orange or 2 melons, tea or coffee.

Evening: Cheese, 6 slices of watermelon or 2 sour apples, grapefruit or 2 oranges or 2,20 lb. melon, tea or coffee without sugar or milk.

Eleventh day

Morning: An egg, 2 breadsticks, 2 tomatoes or a pear, ½ melon or an orange, tea or coffee without sugar or milk.

Evening: Fresh cheese, a heart of lettuce or raw do pepper, 6 slices of watermelon or 2 sour apples, tea or coffee without sugar and milk.

Twelfth day

Morning: 2 eggs, tomato or an apple, a slice of toast or 2 breadsticks, a grapefruit or 2 oranges or 2,20 lb. of melon, tea or coffee without sugar or milk.

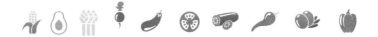

Evening: A cup of 4 milk, 6 slices of watermelon or 4 raw roots, an orange or half a melon, tea or coffee without sugar or milk.

Thirteenth day

Morning: Fresh cheese, raw lettuce or pepper, tomato or an apple, an orange or 2 melon, tea or coffee.

Evening: 2 eggs, a slice of toast, 2 tomatoes, or an apple. an orange or 2 grapefruit or 2,20 lb. of watermelon, tea, or coffee without sugar or milk.

Fourteenth day

Morning: An egg, 6 slices of watermelon or 2 raw artichokes or a pepper, an orange or 2 melons, tea or coffee without sugar or milk.

Evening: 12 raw almonds or hazelnuts, 2 pears, an orange or 2 grapefruit, or 2,20 lb. of melon, tea, or coffee without sugar or milk

Fifteenth day

Morning: 2 eggs, tomato or an apple, 6 slices of watermelon or 2 raw cabbage, an orange or 2 melons, coffee or tea without sugar or milk.

Evening: Fresh cheese, tomato or 3 radishes, 8 almonds or raw hazelnuts, an orange or 2 melon, tea or coffee without sugar or milk.

For the 16th, 17th and 18th day repeat the first three

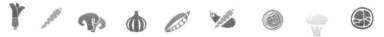

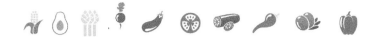

Depending on the results, the aforementioned regime can be repeated two or three times a year with no danger or minimal damage to the subject.

It is preferable to do it in the summer because with it you no longer suffer from the heat.

It is useful to occasionally take a few teaspoons of heavy magnesia.

Eggs are preferable raw, but never cooked with fat.

Diet for the gouty

Do not use industrial sugar.

Excellent purées and soups without aromas of spices.

Milk is good to stretch it a little water.

Raw naturism, heals completely if done on time.

Diet, for those suffering from eczema

Eczema is generally caused by unsuitable nutrition, meat foods, and fish, in particular, dried Scarlet legumes, while green ones and raw vegetables are very good.

Of the cereals exclude oats.

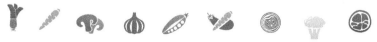

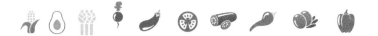

Ban coffee, and take tea very lightly.

No complicated sauces, cheeses, sweets, pastries, fresh bread, canned foods, or sterile in any way.

Going on a raw naturist diet is the best remedy.

Diabetic diet

Good eggs. Exclude starch and replace them with many vegetable fats and cream to obtain the calories of the former.

Many vegetables, preferably raw.

The crushed almonds and oilseeds, put in dishes, both soup and salted, etc., are excellent for replacing cereals and legumes.

Gluten-free bread and pasta; and when it is tolerated, take also rye bread or even almond flour and plasmon.

Zucchini and the whole raw cabbage family are recommended, especially if served plain and seasoned with oil and lemon.

Good chocolate made with sugar-cocoa.

Vermifuge diet

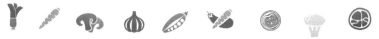

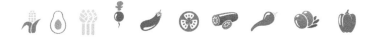

First of all purge with a vegetable purgative, and then every morning, fasting, for four days, give half a tablespoon of the following decoction: 2 oz. of Santolina herbs boiled in three cups of water and collected in two thirds.

The food will be made from toast rubbed with a little garlic and soaked in lemon juice, oil, salt, and parsley, a little green legume puree, fresh fruit, and well-ground oily fruit.

Double portion for adults.

Diet for the old men

All vegetarian eating is excellent, especially raw (see Appendix), as long as you choose things not to chew too much, avoiding irritants: pepper, mustards, cayenne, spices and aromas, substances with cooked acids, condiments, and complicated sauces.

Limit starchy, possibly toasted bread and never fresh bread, better raw bread. Mashed cereal flours and green legumes are excellent, as well as ripe fruit with soft pulp, oily ones must be pounded and eaten immediately.

Avoid fried vegetables and well-cooked dried legumes.

Pastry shops, sweets, and over-rich puddings should be limited. Light tea and cocoa are excellent drinks.

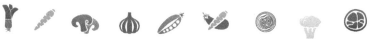

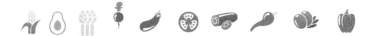

Diet to gain weight

To all dishes rich in starchy or fat add plenty of sweet fruit.

Go to bed early and get up early with a good breakfast with butter, honey, and abundant fresh fruit.

Diet for constipated

Naturism is the best regime, but if you want to limit yourself to vegetarianism, just add a plate of prunes, both fresh and dried, waxed in water, to your common meals, adjusting the quantity with your experience according to the grade of constipation from which one suffers and of individual tolerance.

Raw almonds are also excellent and all cucurbits, possibly raw, are indicated.

Diet for stomach sufferers

The raw food regime, if done with perseverance and discernment, completely puts in order the organism sacrificed by our personal and atavistic errors.

It is not possible to give precise data valid for all people, since each organism has particular tolerances and idiosyncrasies.

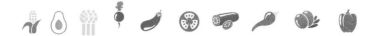

The interesting thing is to abolish cooking. Through cooking, in addition to killing most of the vitamins and all of the biogeny x, chemical combinations still well-known occur, which alter and create harmful sub-products.

Let's see for example the tomato, which while raw is an excellent dissolving, vitalizing, and highly digestible vegetable. cooked it produces uric acids, dyspepsia, liver stones, etc.

So go on a raw regime by choosing and distributing food with your own experience.

Even sick with some gastric diseases considered incurable up to now, they recover completely with the raw food diet.

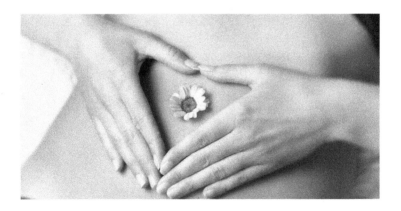

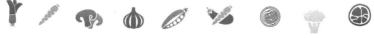

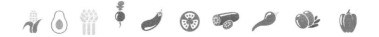

Rational way of distributing meals

Known which are the elements necessary for our nutrition, namely: carbohydrates, proteins (egg whites), mineral salts, fats, cellulose, vitamins, and biogenesis x, and we know that we have them all in the natural products, now let's see how to distribute them harmoniously throughout the day.

In the morning it is useful to take something that prepares us well for the hard work, both manual and mental; and for this purpose, a light revitalizing and dynamogenic meal with nutrient substances of a little volume and which do not require excessive digestive work is indicated. It can be excellently made up of some raw fruit or vegetables: tomato, watermelon, melon, or seed fruit such as almonds, walnuts, hazelnuts, etc. to give the energetic-vitalizing action.

You can add some light protein food with milk, bread and butter, jams and honey, and some stimulants such as coffee, tea, or cocoa, lightly and in small doses.

At noon, when we need to repair the exhausted organism with work, a complete diet is necessary, which can consist of the first course of soup, or dry pasta or timbale, to supply ourselves mainly with carbon hydrates and then a partition to draw on the mineral salts, the cellulose, and the fat.

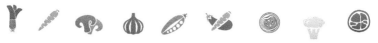

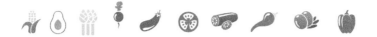

A few more proteins, besides that part we took in the first one, can be ingested with a main dish or with eggs, cheese or dessert.

It is good to remember that our organism does not need more than 30 oz. 1,8of protein per day and more is harmful.

With fruit we complete the meal by drawing a large part of it vitalizing, sugar in its best form, cellulose, dissolving acids, etc.

Around 5 am, especially for those who work very mentally, a cup of tea or light coke is a refreshment.

The raw food in the evening enough to refresh oneself without loading the stomach, it being very hygienic to go to bed to let the body rest as completely as possible and that is without giving it the task of laborious digestion.

A puree, some vegetables or salad, and a few plates of light sauce would be enough pastry, without ever omitting fruit.

All raw food is even better.

For those who love a more thrifty diet either for economic reasons, or because they are more attracted to mental or spiritual life, already knowing that it is very sufficient to fully nourish themselves (and certainly more hygienically than with cooked foods) a piece of black bread is enough, a raw egg

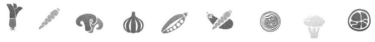

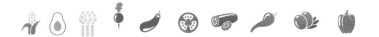

or some fresh milk, and assorted fruit with oil seeds (walnuts, almonds, peanuts, hazelnuts, etc.).

It is also possible to combine modest and complete meals as follows: in the morning bread and fruit or green vegetables (cucumber, tomato, onion, melon, etc.), or a bowl of fresh milk; at noon a soup or a raw egg, a salad or a raw vegetable and mixed fruit; in the evening a slice of raw cheese and fruit.

In all ways, it is always good to vary because the repetition of food tires us.

The multiplicity of differences make the complete and in the alternatives, the organism finds rest and the choice of various small elements.

It is also good to follow what the seasons provide us in more abundance and inexpensively because this too has reason to be.

Let's see, for example, how acidic and juicy fruit abounds in the strong summer heat which refreshes us, and supplies us with replacement fluids, while in winter oilseeds and dried fruit give us calories and more energetic nourishment.

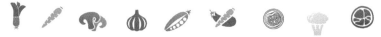

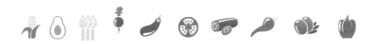

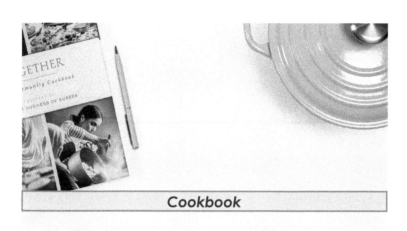

Cookbook

The doses of each formula are generally for six people

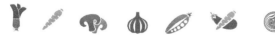

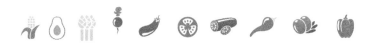

Soups

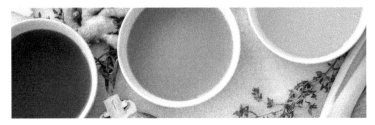

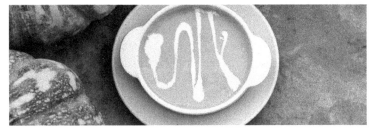

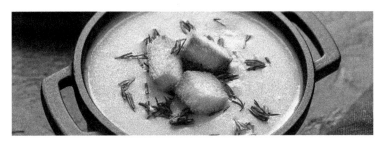

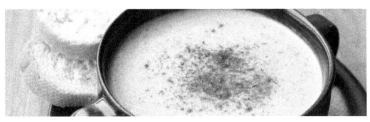

       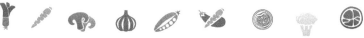

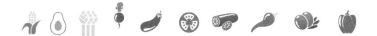

Neapolitan soup

Slice 17,50 oz. of bread marrow and put it in water;

after half an hour, get it out and squeeze it.

Mix it with 7 oz. of grated cheese, 4 hard egg yolks, chopped parsley, salt, and pepper.

Put everything together with as many egg whites as needed to make a not too soft pasta, form it in the plates, and when ready to serve, throw in some broth above the balls that you will flour and fry.

Prepare the broth with this method:

Boil a tablespoon of rice in 1 gal. (US) of water, and add in a small quantity for each: lettuce or escarole, dried peas, torsos, a small cabbage, carrots, celery, parsley, onion, and a tomato; grind everything well and cook slowly for 4 hours.

Add a little salt and color with a little burnt sugar or caramel, filtering it in a towel.

Portuguese soup

Take small sandwiches, grate the rind, uncover them, empty the marrow and fill them with mushroom and walnut filling.

Prepare the filling of mushrooms and walnuts in this way:

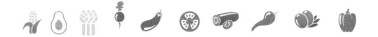

roasted 2 onions well shredded in butter and just golden, throw in 0,70 oz. of dried mushrooms that were cured in water for an hour and shredded and 12 walnuts pounded, adding two bay leaves, nutmeg, pepper, parsley, and salt.

Cook a little and drop.

Apart from soaking. 3,5 oz of bread marrow in milk and put it on the fire, stirring until a batter is formed in which you will pour the first seasoning cold.

Remove the bay leaves and add 4 egg yolks. Mix vigorously.

Use it for fillings.

Put the lid back on, dip them in milk, flour them, pass them in the beaten egg, then in breadcrumbs, and fry them. Arrange them on plates and when ready to serve, pour the broth on top.

Prepare the broth with this method:

boil a tablespoon of rice in 1 gal. (US) of water, and add in a small quantity for each: lettuce or escarole, dried peas, torsos, a small cabbage, carrots, celery, parsley, onion, and a tomato; grind everything well and cook slowly for 4 hours.

Add a little salt and color with a little burnt sugar or caramel, filtering it in a towel.

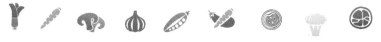

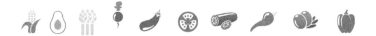

Breadcrumbs Soup

Take 51 fl. Oz. of broth.

Prepare the broth with this method:

boil a tablespoon of rice in 1 gal. (US) of water, and add in a small quantity for each: lettuce or escarole, dried peas, torsos, a small cabbage, carrots, celery, parsley, onion, and tomato.

Grind everything well and cook slowly for 4 hours.

Add a little salt and color with a little burnt sugar or caramel, filtering it in a towel.

Then put half of it in a saucepan, pour in 3,5 oz. of breadcrumbs, and cook over low heat;

when cooked, add a beaten whole egg, a good quantity of grated parmesan cheese and let it bind, adding the rest of the broth, to make a soup with the density you like;

 serve with a piece of fresh butter or 3,40 fl. oz. of cream.

Genoese soup

Boil 17,50 oz. of borage and spinach.

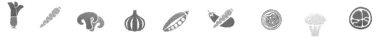

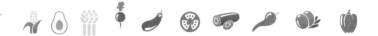

As soon as they are cooked, drain, then crush or finely chop them, pour them into a saucepan with onion, herbs, a pinch of herbs, salt, and pepper, and cook for half an hour.

After cooled, add 5 whole eggs, 1,8 oz. of grated parmesan cheese and cook in a bain-marie.

When this mixture has stiffened, sort it out and put it into small pieces in the broth just before serving.

Prepare the broth with this method:

boil a tablespoon of rice in 1 gal. (US) of water, and add in a small quantity for each: lettuce or escarole, dried peas, torsos, a small cabbage, carrots, celery, parsley, onion, and a tomato;

grind everything well and cook slowly for 4 hours.

Add a little salt and color with a little burnt sugar or caramel, filtering it in a towel.

Cresa soup

Cook well 2,20 lb. of beets and 3 large onions salt, pepper and served.

Melt some butter with a spoonful of flour and a pinch of salt, slowly dilute with 17 fl. oz. US) of hot water and pour the above mixture, and beaten 4 eggs.

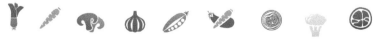

Serve on plates by throwing on them some slices of buttered toast.

Condè Soup

Cook 11 oz. of red beans with salt, a pinch of bicarbonate of soda, and 2 or 3 onions.

Add some broth to 17 fl. oz. (US)

Prepare the broth with this method:

boil a tablespoon of rice in 1 gal. (US) of water, and add in a small quantity for each: lettuce or escarole, dried peas, torsos, a small cabbage, carrots, celery, parsley, onion, and a tomato;

grind everything well and cook slowly for 4 hours.

Add a little salt and color with a little burnt sugar or caramel, filtering it in a towel.

by adding a piece of butter.

Serve on top of toasted or fried bread croutons.

Aurora Soup

Onions 4,40 lb., Butter oz. 7, flour oz. 9, 0,50 gal. (us) milk, 3 egg yolks.

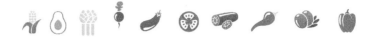

Make to roast, in 3,5 oz. of butter, finely chopped onions, and mix in the flour.

As soon as you see them brown, add them to the milk, stirring vigorously.

Boil for half an hour, get off the heat, and pour in the three egg yolks.

Serve with toasted bread cut into cubes.

Pseudo-clam soup with marinara

The courgette flowers have a special taste that is very reminiscent of seafood and especially clams or clams.

So sauté with 2 large cloves, 2 minced cloves of garlic, nice celery, finely chopped parsley in 5 tablespoons of excellent oil, and when it is well roasted, dilute with 17 fl. oz. (US) of water and boil until the celery is well cooked. Separately boiled in 34 fl. oz. (US) of water and salt;

18 oz. of courgette flowers cut into small pieces and you will melt a pinch of toasted and pounded saffron and a good pinch of salt.

As soon as they are cooked, mix in the sauce and boil again.

Serve with toasted bread or fried cubes.

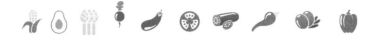

Almond soup

1 oz. of almonds, 34 of 34 fl. oz. US) of milk, ¼ of 8,5 oz. of mozzarella, 1 oz. of butter.

1 tablespoon of flour, 1 onion, 1 half peel the almonds in hot water and finely chop them;

boil them slowly for an hour in 0,50 gal. (US) of milk with the onion and the white part of the celery, remove the onion and celery, mix the flour with the butter and add the rest of the milk and a little pepper and salt.

Stir on the fire until it boils for a few minutes; add the mozzarella again and when it boils again, serve immediately with toasted or fried bread cubes.

Pseudo-frog soup

Sauté with 3 onions, a bunch of chopped carrots, celery and parsley, and brown well in 1,8 oz. of butter and 50 of excellent olive oil.

Moisten with a little wine and after cooking pass through a sieve.

Add the purée to 51 fl. oz. of water with a little salt, add 1 oz. of dried mushrooms cured for an hour in water and chopped, another bunch of carrots with a few celery leaves, garlic, and a pinch of spices.

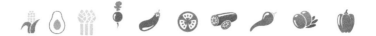

Boil for half an hour and serve by throwing a handful on each plate of diced fried bread.

Soup of pseudo-clams

Make it like that of pseudo-frogs, adding 7 oz. of shredded pumpkin flower (whose pollen has the taste of seafood), and a pinch of toasted and pulverized saffron.

Serve with fried bread cubes.

Celery soup

6 celery hearts, 2 carrots, 2 onions, a cabbage (all well chopped), and 0,50 gal. (US) of water. Butter 2 oz.

Fry the onion in butter, pour in the water, and boil with the vegetables for an hour, adding pepper and salt.

Serve with fried croutons and buffed cheese.

British soap

Two heads of celery, 3,5 oz. of butter, 34 fl. oz. US) of water, salt and white pepper, 2 egg yolks, 1 gal. (US) of milk, and 3,40 fl. oz. of mozzarella.

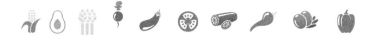

Melt the butter, fry the celery and mix well. Pour in the water and boil until cooked.

Go down and go to the sieve.

Return to the saucepan with the milk and stir until it boils. Whisk the eggs and cream in a bowl and pour over the boiling liquid.

Serve with or without butter croutons.

Mountain soup

Cut some good mushrooms into small pieces of one centimeter and grind a couple of black truffles.

Throw them in 34 fl. oz. (US) of broth.

Prepare the broth with this method:

boil a tablespoon of rice in 1 gal. (US) of water, and add in a small quantity for each: lettuce or escarole, dried peas, torsos, a small cabbage, carrots, celery, parsley, onion, and a tomato;

grind everything well and cook slowly for 4 hours.

Add a little salt and color with a little burnt sugar or caramel, filtering it in a towel.

Them boil for half an hour.

Arrange six slices of fried bread in six soup plates and sprinkle with Parmesan cheese.

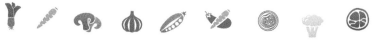

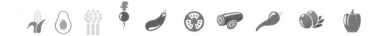

Blend 3 whole eggs with a pinch of salt, chopped parsley, herbs, and pepper.

Remove the broth from the heat and let it cool a little, to mix in the beaten eggs.

Put it back on the heat, always stirring and when a little tied up pour it into the plates.

White soup

Milk 0,50 gal. (US), parmesan cheese 5,30 oz., 4 eggs, bread 11 oz., large onions 3.

Take a little butter and fry the chopped onions.

Just lightly browned, pour in a stir or two of milk, boil for 10 minutes, and pass through the sieve.

Return to the saucepan, pouring the rest of the milk, waiting for it to boil.

Cut the bread into slices and toast it, place it in the soup bowl in layers, wetting it with the beaten eggs, and sprinkling it each time with grated parmesan cheese.

Pour over the boiling milk where you have put some salt and serve.

Hard pan soup with tomato

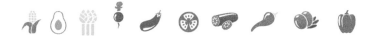

Hardpan 2,20 lb., tomatoes 4,40 lb., onions 2, butter 3,5 oz., garnished bunch.

Put the hard bread in water and when it is very soft. remove the crust; squeeze it and pass it through a sieve; wash and puree the raw tomato.

Aside, roast the finely chopped onion in butter and throw in both the bread and the tomato sauce, adding the garnished bunch, and cook by pouring a little water if necessary.

Finally, add salt, spices, and a spoonful of butter to serve immediately.

Mushroom soup

Take 4,40 lb. of good mushrooms, cut them, wash them and add some truffles into small pieces.

Separately, knot 6 onions cut in quarters in a diaper, 2 chopped tomatoes, 2 bay leaves, small pieces of orange peel, and 4 cloves;

put everything in a saucepan with salt, pepper, a good pinch of pulverized saffron, chopped parsley, and 0,50 gal. (US) of dry white wine.

Add a 2 spoon of oil, 34 fl. oz. US) of water, where you have dissolved 2 teaspoons of starch.

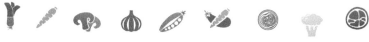

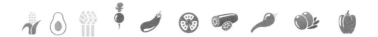

Cook for an hour. remove the bag of herbs and serve on the plates where you have placed a couple of slices of toast.

Milk and egg soup

Boil 1. 12 of milk adding a little salt.

Bind with 6 egg yolks.

As soon as it is thick, it should be served with toasted and buttered croutons.

Bean soup with celery

Take 21 oz. of white beans and put them in water, possibly the night before.

Add a pinch of bicarbonate of soda, water and cook slowly.

Halfway through cooking, remove the skins and add celery and carrots cut into small pieces.

When they are completely cooked, add some good olive oil, a little pepper, and serve.

Italian vegetable soap

Cook separately 7 oz. of white beans and when they are almost cooked, set them aside.

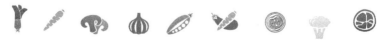

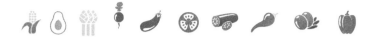

In another saucepan, cook carrots, celery, leeks, broccoli, and all those vegetables of the time that you like best with a little water.

When this mixture is almost cooked, add beans and 9 oz. of rice, salt, pepper, and oil or butter, whichever you prefer.

Cook everything, adding water when needed. It is served hot or cold, sprinkling or not with parmesan.

Pasta with lentils (Soup)

Cook 14 oz. of lentils in water with salt and remove them; heat and drop the pasta (stars, penne, sparrow tongue, etc.).

Pour yourself some good olive oil, a pinch of pepper, and when it is well cooked served.

If desired, it is seasoned with butter or mozzarella.

Pasta with beans (Soup)

Cook 14 oz. of beans in water with salt and remove them; heat and drop the pasta (stars, penne, sparrow tongue, etc.).

Pour yourself some good olive oil, a pinch of pepper, and when it is well cooked served.

If desired, it is seasoned with butter or mozzarella.

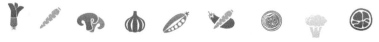

Pasta with dried broad beans

Cook 14 oz. of dried broad beans in water with salt and remove them;

heat and drop the pasta (stars, penne, sparrow tongue, etc.

Pour yourself some good olive oil, a pinch of pepper, and when it is well cooked served.

If desired, it is seasoned with butter or mozzarella.

Pasta with broccoli (Soup)

Cut nice broccoli into small pieces and boil it in water.

When it is almost cooked, add the pasta (stars, penne, sparrow tongue, etc.), add oil, salt, pepper.

When cooked, served.

This too can be done better by bypassing the broccoli through a sieve and seasoning with butter or mozzarella.

Pasta with green beans

Peel twice 2,20 lb. of green beans and put them to cook in water.

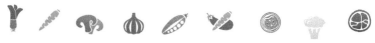

When unpacked throw 14,40 lb. of pasta of your choice seasoned with salt, pepper, oil, or butter.

Oriental soup

Slowly rain 6 tablespoons of tapioca or sagou into 0,50 gal. (US) of broth or cold milk, stirring constantly.

Prepare the broth with this method:

boil a tablespoon of rice in 1 gal. (US) of water, and add in a small quantity for each: lettuce or escarole, dried peas, torsos, a small cabbage, carrots, celery, parsley, onion, and a tomato.

Grind everything well and cook slowly for 4 hours.

Add a little salt and color with a little burnt sugar or caramel, filtering it in a towel.

Then put on the fire without leaving stirring.

In about 20 minutes it will be cooked.

Before serving, add a knob of butter and salt.

Spring soup

Green peas 1 lb.; green beans 1 lb.; rice 3,5 oz.; carrots 4; celery 1; parsley - 1 bunch; onion 1; butter 1,8 oz.

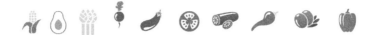

Lightly brown the well-chopped onion in the butter and add the peas, the broad beans shelled twice, the finely chopped carrots, with water, salt, and pepper.

Cook for half an hour, then add the rice and as soon as it is cooked, serve with or without the cheese.

Munich soup

Make nice thin slices of bread equal in shape, and thickness, toast them on the grill, spread with butter and sprinkle with a little fine sugar;

arrange them on a plate and pour over 51fl.oz of boiling milk with a pinch of salt.

If you want, tie the milk with some egg yolks before pouring it.

Mock-turtle soup

Take 17 fl. oz. (US) of broth.

Prepare the broth with this method:

boil a tablespoon of rice in 1 gal. (US) of water, and add in a small quantity for each: lettuce or escarole, dried peas, torsos, a small cabbage, carrots, celery, parsley, onion, and a tomato;

grind everything well and cook slowly for 4 hours.

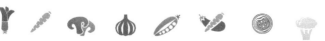

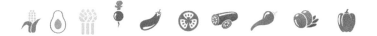

Add a little salt and color with a little burnt sugar or caramel, filtering it in a towel.

Then add, tied in a diaper, a bunch of parsley, thyme, sage, basil, onion, 2 cloves, 2 bay leaves, pepper, salt, and grated nutmeg.

Cook for a good hour.

Add some mushrooms and some truffles into small pieces, diluted with water where you have dissolved a good spoonful of potato starch.

Pour in a glass of old white wine, the sauce of half a lemon, and a pinch of cayenne pepper.

Cook for another half hour, put some hard egg yolks inside.

Leave the aromas knot and serve with fried diced croutons.

Austrian soup

9 Oz. of black beans, 1,7 oz. of German barley, 2 onions, 3 3 cloves, 2 whole pimientos (hot peppers), 9 oz. of carrots, 6 strands of celery, 50 g of butter.

Put the beans in the water a little earlier.

Cut the onions and fry in the butter; drain the beans and put everything to boil in 0,50 gal. (US) of water.

Cook for 4 hours adding hot water as needed.

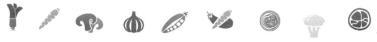

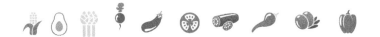

Then pass everything through a sieve and season with finely chopped parsley, majorana, pepper, and salt.

You can also serve it with diced fried croutons.

Housewife soup

Beans 200 gr, 1 cabbage, 100 g carrots, green beans 300 g of green beans, 200 g of pasta, 250 g of potatoes, 50 g of butter and oil, parsley, and herbs.

Two dishes are made with the above ingredients.

Boil the dried broad beans in 1 gal. (US) of water and when they are cooked add all the vegetables, except the potatoes, and season with salt, pour everything, and keep the broth.

Take a fried with oil, butter, chopped onion and toss the potatoes they making them a get brown.

Pour in the legume broth and when it boils add the pasta, parsley, and spices.

With the cooked legumes you will make a cold salad that you can also dress with mayonnaise, capers, gherkins, etc. adding lettuce or cucumber or other raw seasonal vegetables.

Polenta soup with subisso

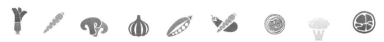

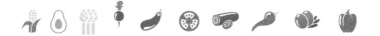

Polenta or corn semolina 9 oz., 34 fl. oz. of milk, butter 5,30 oz., onion 5,30 oz.

Roast the onion in 3,5 oz of butter and just golden brown put the polenta, stirring for 3 minutes always on the fire.

Then slowly pour in the milk and then just enough water.

Add salt, pepper and stir continuously for half an hour. Throw in the rest of the butter and if you want it tastier, mix 3,5 oz. of mozzarella and serve immediately.

Chilean lentils

Lentils 250 oz., butter 3,5 oz., olive oil 1,8 oz., seat 1, cayenne, 2 onions and 6 tomatoes.

Chop the onions, and tomatoes from which you have first removed the peel, and seeds, and make a good fried with butter and oil.

Cook the lentils in water with a pinch of bicarbonate of soda.

Add the chopped celery, the cayenne pepper (if you like) and when well cooked, tighten them together with the sauté.

You can serve them as a soup by putting some toasted bread into cubes.

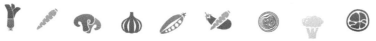

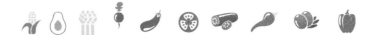

Maggiolina soup

A small cabbage, 3,5 oz. carrots, 7 oz. of green beans, 3,5 oz. of rice, 9 oz. of potatoes, 7 oz. of zucchini, 3,5 oz. of torsos, 7 oz. of peeled peas, celery, parsley, basil, onion, butter, and oil.

Being all stuff of equal cooking time, put everything, chopped, in a saucepan with 17 fl. oz. (US)s of water, salt, pepper, spices, 1,8 oz. of butter and the same of excellent oil.

Cook over low heat, never stirring, and when the rice is cooked, descend and serve.

Chilean-style beans

Boil 28 oz. of white beans in 1 gal. (US) of water, a pinch of bicarbonate of soda and more with salt.

When almost cooked, strain them by throwing away the water.

Fry 2 onions in 3,40 fl. oz. of oil or 3,5 oz. of butter and add the beans.

Cook pouring a little water at a time and season with salt and cayenne pepper.

Soup house

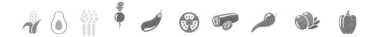

A small cabbage, 3,5 oz. carrots, 7 oz. of green beans, 3,5 oz. of rice, 9 oz. of potatoes, 7 oz. of zucchini, 3,5 oz. of torsos, 7 oz.of peeled peas, celery, parsley, basil, onion, butter, and oil.

Being all stuff of equal cooking time, put everything, chopped, in a saucepan with 51 fl. oz. of water, salt, pepper, spices, 1,8 oz. of butter and the same of excellent oil.

Cook over low heat, never stirring, and when the rice is cooked, descend and serve.

adding on the plate, before serving, 6 to 8 cubes of a square centimeter of fresh cheese, pouring the boiling soup over it.

Breaded soup

Breadcrumbs marinated 4,6 oz.; 4 eggs; parmesan 1,8 oz., flavorings.

Make a mixture of the aforesaid ingredients and dilute with lukewarm broth.

Prepare the broth with this method:

boil a tablespoon of rice in 1 gal. (US) of water, and add in a small quantity for each: lettuce or escarole, dried peas, torsos, a small cabbage, carrots, celery, parsley, onion, and a tomato;

grind everything well and cook slowly for 4 hours.

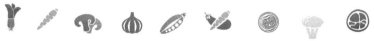

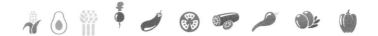

Add a little salt and color with a little burnt sugar or caramel, filtering it in a towel.

Cook it over very low heat, taking care to detach what adheres to the walls.

When it has thickened, serve.

You can add peas or other vegetables that you will cook separately.

Sour Potato Soup

Potatoes 4,40 lb., butter 3,5 oz., large onions 3, flour 3,5 oz., 2 lemons, herbs, and 6 walnuts.

Peel and dice the potatoes by putting them in water. Separately, finely chop the onions and lightly brown them in half the butter, then throw in the flour, and always stirring, dilute with water, avoiding the clumping of the flour.

Throw in the poured potatoes, a good pinch of salt 'and stirring again add water as required.

When they are cooked, add the other half of the butter, the lemon juice and serve by sowing them with the chopped herb and the pounded walnuts.

Passatelle in Italian-style soup

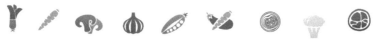

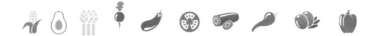

Eggs 3, grated cheese 1,8 oz., breadcrumbs 1 oz., pounded walnuts 1 oz.. Knead everything together and pass from a device or a cup like a syringe.

Cook in broth.

Prepare the broth with this method:

boil a tablespoon of rice in 1 gal. (US) of water, and add in a small quantity for each: lettuce or escarole, dried peas, torsos, a small cabbage, carrots, celery, parsley, onion, and a tomato;

grind everything well and cook slowly for 4 hours.

Add a little salt and color with a little burnt sugar or caramel, filtering it in a towel.

Duxellese soup

Small cabbage 1, carrots 4, butter 7 oz. ; 34 fl. oz.US) milk.

Leeks 6, onions 3, flour 5,30 oz., pepper and salt.

Finely chop all the vegetables and cook them with 34 fl. oz. US) of water and half the butter.

As soon as they boil, count half an hour and then pour half the milk in which you have dissolved the flour in porridge.

Leave to cook for another 10 minutes, always stirring, then descend from the heat and season with salt,

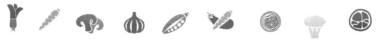

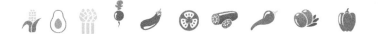

pepper, the other half of the butter and the rest of the milk.

Serve immediately with or without croutons.

Green soup

Cook in 51 fl. oz. of water until 180 g of peeled peas have dissolved, add 7 oz.. of chopped spinach, 1 bunch of aromatic herbs, chopped onion, a clove of garlic, and two slices of bread fried in butter.

Boil again for half an hour and pass through a sieve.

Place the liquid in a saucepan bringing the liquid to 0.50 gal. (USA) and when it boils add a very small paste to your taste in the quantity of 4 tablespoons;

Season with salt and pepper and, when cooked, add a piece of butter and serve.

Varied green soup

A bunch of chard, 1 lettuce, 1 bunch of spinach, a quarter of a cabbage, or 1 small cabbage.

Chop everything up.

Fry with a piece of butter, chopped onion, and all the smells you like best.

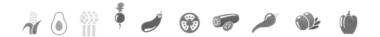

Throw in the well-soaked herbs together with 2 sliced potatoes and some chopped tomatoes.

Add salt, pepper and cook adding water until everything is well undone.

Then sieve, bring to 0,50 gal. (US), season with butter, and cook rice or pasta or tapioca in it.

London soup

One cabbage, 1 bunch of carrots, 4 leeks, 2 large onions, 2 sedans1, 1 teaspoon of vinegar, 3.5 oz. of butter, 5.30 oz. of rice, a bay leaf, a pinch of oregano, thyme, majorana, pepper, salt, 2 teaspoons of curry, 3.5 oz. of mozzarella, 1 pound of apples, and a teaspoon of lemon juice.

Fry the onion in butter with the apples, cut into cubes, then add the chopped vegetables, curry, rice, and aromatic herbs; when the butter is absorbed, 0,50 gal. (US) of water are added and it is boiled for two hours.

Before serving, pour in the cream and lemon juice.

Julian soup

Prepare 0,50 gal. (US) of broth in this method:

boil a tablespoon of rice in 1 gal. (US) of water, and add in a small quantity for each: lettuce or escarole,

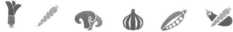

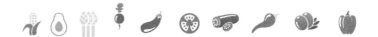

dried peas, torsos, a small cabbage, carrots, celery, parsley, onion, and tomato; grind everything well and cook slowly for 4 hours.

Add a little salt and color with a little burnt sugar or caramel, filtering it in a towel.

When it boils, throw in 7 oz. of potatoes, 7 oz. of carrots, 3,5 oz. of cabbage, 2 hearts of celery, parsley, and herbs cut into thin strips.

When cooked, serve with fried croutons on the side.

English macaroni soup

7 oz. of cabbage, oz. 7 of carrots, oz. 7 of onions, parsley, 0,50 gal. (us) milk, butter oz. 3, broken macaroni or penne 9 oz.

Chop the vegetables and boil them in 34 fl. oz. US) of water with salt and a little pepper.

When they are almost cooked, add the milk, the macaroni, the chopped parsley and cook while stirring.

Add the butter and serve.

Leek soup

Leeks 14 oz., potatoes 1lb., 1 heart of celery, 2 oz. of butter.

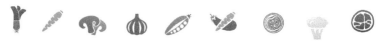

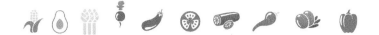

Shred and fry in butter with pepper and salt.

Add 0,50 gal. (US) of water.

Boil for 112 hours. Serve with fried diced croutons.

Egyptian lens soup

11 Oz. of lentils, 2 chopped cubes, 17 fl. Oz. of milk, ½ teaspoon of curry, and pepper.

Keeping the lentils in the water for a few hours.

Cook them with the onion in enough water to cover them and then pass through the sieve.

Melt 1,8 oz. of flour in milk, mix everything with curry, squeeze and serve with croutons.

Soup of lentils and rice

Put in water for a few hours 11 oz. of lentils and then boil them in 0,50 gal. (US) of water;

when cooked put inside 3,5 oz. of rice, 2 onions, 3 chopped carrots and parsley, salt, pepper, and a pinch of bicarbonate alone.

Before serving, pour 3,40 fl. oz. of mozzarella.

English milk soup

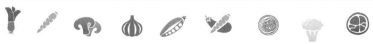

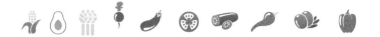

Three-quarters of a 34 fl. oz. US) of broth in this method:

boil a tablespoon of rice in 1 gal. (US) of water, and add in a small quantity for each: lettuce or escarole, dried peas, torsos, a small cabbage, carrots, celery, parsley, onion, and a tomato;

grind everything well and cook slowly for 4 hours.

Add a little salt and color with a little burnt sugar or caramel, filtering it in a towel.

250 Oz. of potatoes, 1 onion, 2 carrots, a little celery.

Boil the broth and throw in the well-cut and cut vegetables.

When cooked, pass the sieve and put it back on the heat adding the milk.

As soon as it boils, serve with diced fried bread.

Mushroom soup

1 lb. of fresh mushrooms or 5,30 oz. of the dry ones marinated in water for at least 1 hour, 34 of 34 fl. Oz. of vegetable broth.

Prepare the broth with this method:

boil a tablespoon of rice in 1 gal. (US) of water, and add in a small quantity for each: lettuce or escarole,

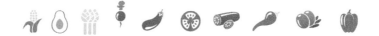

dried peas, torsos, a small cabbage, carrots, celery, parsley, onion, and a tomato;

grind everything well and cook slowly for 4 hours.

Add a little salt and color with a little burnt sugar or caramel, filtering it in a towel.

34 fl. oz. US) of milk.

Cut the mushrooms into slices and cook them in the broth until they become tender.

Fry separately 3,5 oz. of sliced carrots in 2,5 oz. of butter.

Combine everything with the milk where you have dissolved a little starch, and serve with croutons.

Ricotta soup

Roast a large onion in 2 oz. of butter without becoming dark, moisten it with a glass of dry white wine, and just blended pulp 7 oz. of ricotta.

Extend with 17 fl. oz. (US) of milk and 1 gal. (US) of water and salt.

After half an hour of cooking, pass through the sieve, heat, and serve with fried crostini cubes.

Winter Soup

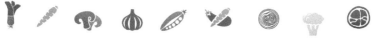

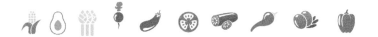

Potatoes 3 lb. 1 34 fl. oz. US) milk, butter 5,30 oz., abundant parsley, 10 walnuts.

Boil the peeled potatoes and pass them one by one, dropping them into the warm milk.

Bind with 4 egg yolks, put salt and pepper, and pour slices of bread fried in butter on plates, sprinkle 10 plague nuts and finely chopped parsley.

Chilean Puchero

Make 17 fl.oz.2 of broth.

Prepare the broth with this method:

boil a tablespoon of rice in 1 gal. (US) of water, and add in a small quantity for each: lettuce or escarole, dried peas, torsos, a small cabbage, carrots, celery, parsley, onion, and a tomato; grind everything well and cook slowly for 4 hours.

Add a little salt and color with a little burnt sugar or caramel, filtering it in a towel.

Boil 6 pieces of soft corn cobs, 6 pieces of pumpkin, 6 onions, a cabbage, 6 potatoes, 6 cabbage, and 6 carrots.

When cooked, divide them into 6 soup plates, pour the broth over them and sprinkle with cheese.

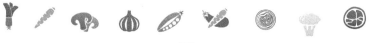

Rumford Soup

Boiled 9 oz. Of pearl barley and 7 oz. of dried shelled peas in 1 gal. (US) of water until well cooked.

Add 14 oz. shredded potatoes, a bunch of herbs, salt, pepper, 3,40 fl. oz. vinegar, a little celery, a few slices of carrot, spring onions, cabbage, or other vegetables to taste.

Extend with water if necessary and serve with croutons.

White beans soup

Boiled white bean soup 14 oz. of white beans with 3 carrots, chopped celery, celery, and parsley in 0,80 gal. (US) of water with a pinch of bicarbonate, adding water if necessary.

Pass through the sieve, lengthened if necessary, put on the fire with a little salt, white pepper, and tie with a little flour dissolved in milk.

As soon as it is thick, pour 3,40 fl. oz. of mozzarella and serve on slices of fried bread.

Green soup

Artichokes 4, oz. 11 of dried or green shelled peas, 2 carrots, a good handful of chopped spinach or nettles, parsley, and onion.

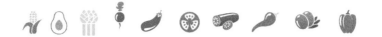

Boil in 0,80 gal. (US) of water adding more if necessary.

When everything is well cooked, strain, heat, and pour 3,40 fl. oz. of cream, served with croutons.

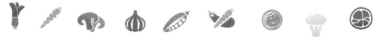

Raw soups

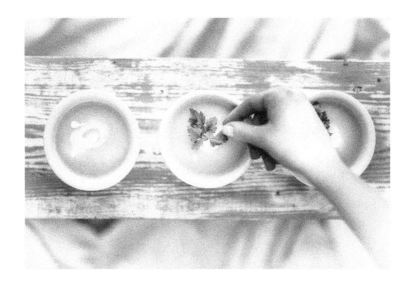

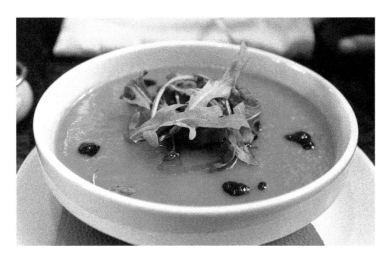

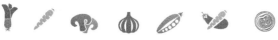

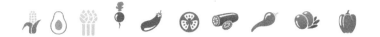

Soup with Corn

Slices 2,20 lb. of tomatoes, 1 cucumber, 2 zucchini, 3 onions;

sprinkle with a little salt, chopped herbs, a small clove of garlic, a pinch of oregano, and pour into a sieve, collecting the sauce for 2 hours.

Then squeeze the rest in the press and add the sauce to the first.

Place on plates and take one green cornbread per portion, to which you will cut the grains (soft milk) with a knife, making them fall into the vegetable broth.

It is a delicious and very nutritious soup if the corn is harvested at the right point.

Raw spring soup

Oranges 2,20 lb., 5,30 oz. of tender peas, 7 oz. of very tender shelled green beans, 2 yellow carrots, onion, oil, and lemon.

Squeeze the oranges and add all the ingredients with the chopped or rasped carrots and the juice of a lemon.

Good chewing is always of paramount importance. When you cannot do it well due to a defect in teeth, you pass everything to a machine.

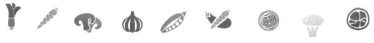

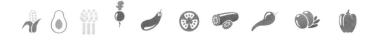

Winter soup

Take 4,40 lb. of giant yellow squash, slice it, sprinkle it with a little salt, and put it to drain on the steak together with 4,40 lb. of sliced onions, 4 carrots, 1 head of celery, 1 garlic, parsley, and 4 sliced pure oranges.

After 2 hours, press and combine the two sauces by dissolving a teaspoon of English mustard and a little fine olive oil.

Protect by sowing 3 pounded walnuts or other oily seeds in each dish.

Cantaloupe soup

Take 2,20 lb. of tomatoes, 7 oz. onions, 1 cocoon, 1 garlic, and chopped parsley.

Mash the tomatoes after they have been well washed, cut the chopped tomatoes and watermelon into thin slices, add the chopped parsley and garlic, sprinkle with a little salt, and put on the steak to drain.

After 2 hours squeeze in the press and combine the two sauces.

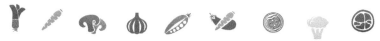

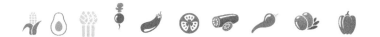

Thinly slice a cantaloupe or similar strong-scented melon and divide it into plates by pouring over the raw broth and 3,40 fl. oz. of mozzarella.

Beetroot soup

Take 2,20 lb. of beets, 4 well washed and sliced carrots together with 3,5 oz. of onions, parsley, 1 clove of garlic, and oregano.

Sprinkle lightly with salt and drain on the sieve for 2 hours. Grind and season the sauce with lemon and oil, sowing walnuts or other ground oily seeds.

Semolina soup

Slice 2 cucumbers or watermelons, 2,20 lb. of tomatoes, and 3,5 oz. of onions;

sprinkle them with a little salt, possibly celery, and put them to drain in the sieve, collecting the sauce.

After 2 hours press them, add the two sauces, pour a lemon beaten with very fine oil and abundant parsley, and distribute it on the plates, mixing in every 2 tablespoons of softened semolina.

Spicy soup for stomach dullers

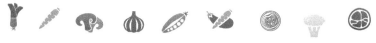

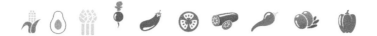

Sliced 4,40 lb. of zucchini, 2 watermelons or 2 cucumbers, 4 carrots, 3,5 oz. of onions, lb. 1 of tomatoes and sprinkle a little salt and oregano.

Leave to make for 2 hours and squeeze the solid in the press. In a small cup, melt 2 teaspoons of yellow English mustard with lemon juice and a little minced garlic put it in the broth, and let it swim a few points of thinly sliced asparagus and carrots or very tender green peas or raw chopped truffles.

Soup with corn

Take 6 corn cobs still tender from milk and cut the grains with a sharp knife.

Put in soup plates pouring raw tomato or orange sauce, celery salt or a little cooking salt, and very fine olive oil.

Fresh tomato soup

Clean well 2,20 lb. of ripe and healthy tomatoes, pass them to the machine and in this sauce add 3 grated carrots, chopped onion, garlic, and fine herbs.

Season with good oil or cream, a little salt, and a few very tender green peas if it is the season.

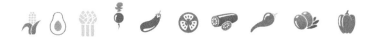

Soup of cereals and dried legumes

Choose what you like and in the proportion of 0,70 oz. per person, put it to macerate in water with a pinch of bicarbonate.

When the seeds are well swollen and tender, which cannot happen for 12 hours, squeeze them.

Rinse them in the living water and pass them to the grinder.

Separately, make a vegetable broth.

Prepare the broth with this method:

tomatoes 3,30 lb., 2 watermelons or cucumbers, 1 onion, a few roots, parsley, and herbs.

Chop everything minutely and sprinkle with a little salt. Let it brew for a couple of hours and squeeze the rest into the small press.

To protect it, place small balls of truffles or raw minced mushrooms or ground oil seeds on the plates.

Squeeze some lemon and add a few drops of olive oil

If you want, you can swim with slices of cantaloupe melon.

You can add or change some vegetables according to the season and taste.

Then divide the macerated seeds and serve with lemon sauce, oil or cream, the rasping of celery root, or very fine parsley to your taste.

Complete tomato soap

Take 2,20 lb. of beautiful tomatoes, peel them, cut them in half horizontally, and remove the seeds, which you will drain to collect the sauce.

Cut the pulp into small pieces and arrange it on plates, sprinkle a little chopped parsley and plenty of chopped parsley, pour in the sauce from the seeds, sprinkle with a little salt if possible celery, sprinkle with ground oil seeds, a little oil, or cream, lemon and 4 tablespoons of oat flakes soaked in water for 6 hours.

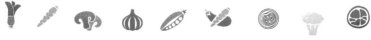

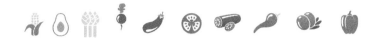

Dear Reader
I am an emerging writer and, with the sales made from the book, I can continue my studies to publish other books on the subject. I would appreciate an honest review from you.

Join Kimberley Smith newsletter to be informed about new books:
kimb.smith.books@gmail.com

Thanks for your support

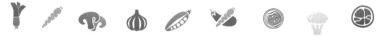

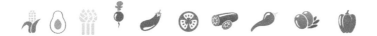

Cover by Bluebird Provisions on Pixabay

Visit the author's page

Write to: kimb.smith.books@gmail.com

OTHER PUBLICATIONS BY KIMBERLEY SMITH:

Raising Chickens For Eggs:

The Beginner's Guide To Building A Chicken-Coop, To Learn How to Raise A Happy Backyard Flock.
A Homesteading Solution While You Are At Home

Hydroponic Gardening:

A Detailed Guide on Hydronics to Learn the Principles Behind Gardening and Build a Wonderful System While at Home. Techniques for Your Vegetable Cultivations

Keto Copycat Cookbook Restaurant:

A Keto Diet to Feel Your Best. Easy Recipes for Beginners for All Seasons From Appetizers to Desserts to Reduce Inflammation, Lose Weight, and Heal the Immune System

EASY KETO DESERTS

67 Recipes for Beginners for All Seasons

to Reduce Inflammation, Lose Weight, And Heal the Immune System

A Ketogenic Diet to Feel Your Best

CPSIA information can be obtained
at www.ICGtesting.com
Printed in the USA
BVHW090224010621
608491BV00011B/2110